Strengthening
the Lower Body

Author and Publisher
Earle E. Liederman
305 Broadway · New York

STRENGTHENING THE LOWER BODY

(ORIGINAL VERSION, RESTORED)

By

EARLE LIEDERMAN

Original Publisher: Earle Liederman, 305 Broadway, New York, 1927

PUBLISHED BY O'Faolain Patriot LLC, Copyright 2011

info@PhysicalCultureBooks.com

ISBN-13: 978-1468015300

ISBN-10: 1468015303

Published in the United States of America

To Order More Copies Visit: Physical Culture Books.com

STRENGTHENING THE LOWER BODY

I WAS giving a series of lectures on physical culture some years ago in Chicago when a young doctor, who was some kind of a teacher in a medical college, took exception to a statement I made concerning the influence of exercise on health.

The doctor, who was pretty well married to the idea that the only way you could get relief from sickness was to take something out of a bottle, or else swallow a couple of pills, said:

"Mr. Liederman, do you mean to say that if a person takes exercise that he won't get sick; or if he is sick, that you can help him to get well by having him take exercises?"

I said: "I don't make any foolish claims to the effect that you can prevent all kinds of sickness by putting the body in perfect physical condition. Nor do I mean to say that all forms of sickness can be overcome by having a man take the right kind of exercises, for there are many kinds of sickness that are the result of direct infection.

"I do mean to say, however, that if a man will put himself into A-1 physical condition by the proper kind of exercises and right living, that he stands a very small chance of ever developing any of the chronic ailments due to disorders of digestion and metabolism and the lack of proper elimination, that constitute nine-tenths of the doctor's business today.

"And I mean further to say, that even if he does contract acute diseases from infection, exposure, or other causes, that he'll get well about five times as fast if he is in fine physical shape as he would if he is all out of condition, from lack of proper physical exercise and failure to observe the essential rules of hygiene which I teach."

The doctor listened to what I had to say, and when I got through, he said: "Mr. Liederman, I take it all back. I see that what you have to say is founded on strict common sense. You win."

And this is now rapidly becoming the attitude of physicians all over the world. They are giving less and less medicine, and paying more and more attention to diet, hygiene, fresh air and exercise. And they're doing their patients infinitely more good than they ever did before, as a consequence.

From the standpoint of health, there is no doubt that the abdominal muscles are the most important of all the muscles in the body—except, of course, the heart muscles. For the condition of the abdominal muscles either makes or mars the function of all the digestive organs, as well as the most important organs of elimination, the bowels.

Strong, well-developed waist muscles, that hold the abdominal organs up in position and that prevent the sagging or prolapse that interferes so disastrously with their function, are absolutely essential to everyone who wants to remain in good health.

Therefore, I urge you to pay particular attention to the development of the muscles of the waist, so that you may enjoy the better health which development of the abdominal muscles brings about.

Now, to the average person the waist consists of two sizes, small and large. To the student of anatomy, however, there are as many variations in the waist as there are faces in the street. There are also long waists and short waists. The longer waisted individual usually has more endurance and more flexibility than a person who has a short waistline. In the trained athlete the waist usually presents its best appearance at about twenty-five years of age, for after that, there is a tendency to accumulate flesh, regardless of what physical training an individual may do.

This change may merely be a gain of an inch or two, but, nevertheless, after twenty-five years of age, the waist is never as small. Before the age of twenty, you very seldom see the muscles of the waist as thoroughly developed as they are after a man has reached his full growth, for, as a rule, the youthful waistline has a tendency to go in at the sides, where the external oblique abdominus muscle lies. Later on, when the boy commences training of the trunk region, the waist assumes a square appearance, owing to the pleasing development of the external oblique muscles.

The first muscle to show its appearance when the student performs a few weeks of abdominal work is the rectus abdominus. This muscle covers the front of the abdominal region, and when highly developed has a washboard appearance of eight fleshy digitations. If not developed to the maximum there are only six showing.

One of the finest examples of abdominal development I have ever seen was that of the late Eugen Sandow. His muscles were of unusual quality and contour and he possessed remarkable control of them. The constant contraction of these abdominal muscles helps greatly to bring them out. The most simple contraction is performed by bending slightly forward and pressing downward on the thighs with the hands. The next step is the isolation of the rectus abdominus.

This is performed by emptying the lungs of air, pressing downward and outward on the upper thighs with the hands, and at the same time drawing in the abdominal wall, causing a cavity on each side of these muscles. I have seen some remarkable controls in this region. The single isolation, that is, having one side of the rectus abdominus muscle contracted and the other side drawn in with the abdominal cavity, is undoubtedly the most phenomenal of any muscular control that can be accomplished.

The quickest way to gain flesh around the abdominal region is to make yourself comfortable, and the larger the waistline becomes the more the skin is placed upon a stretcher, until the weight of the superfluous flesh in front of the waist becomes saggy and lower. It is a simple matter to accumulate extra weight around the waist, but it is a very hard matter to rid oneself of it, as you may possibly have already found out. If a person will be careful of his diet, does not sit too much, and makes a point of standing erect at all times, he need have very little fear of becoming fleshy around the waist, especially if he performs daily sit-ups and trunk movements.

After thirty or thirty-five years of age, fleshy accumulations not only in the front of the waist, but in the sides and back, as well as the hips, will gradually form rolls of fat that are much harder to get rid of than is the superfluous flesh that gathers in front of the waist. A person whose habits are sedentary must pay special attention to the side of his back, the side of his waist and the front of his abdomen, if he expects to retain a small waistline the remainder of his days. He also must be careful of his diet, if he is inclined to put on flesh.

The nervous type individual who is high-strung need have little fear of ever acquiring a large waist, and should be thankful for that reason. If, however, he will devote care and attention to the rest of his body, combined with systematic training, he will find his progress much easier, and will waste less energy in his progress than the person who has constantly to fight the accumulation of flesh around the abdomen. My idea of the type of waist an athlete should possess is square, well-developed and yet slim, at the same time long, thus giving one remarkable endurance, flexibility and perfectly functioning organs.

It is very difficult to set a standard of measurements for the waistline, for a great deal depends upon the height and frame-work of the individual. A person who has a large frame-work, naturally

will have a much wider waist than his small-boned competitor. This width of the waist will naturally increase the size by a couple of inches. The smaller the waist is, the larger the chest appears, and the broader the shoulders look. A person who devotes a lot of attention to abdominal work need never have any fear of constipation, indigestion or other similar ailments so common to the ordinary public.

As I said before, the waistline to the obese individual is one of the most stubborn parts of the body to reduce, especially if considerable superfluous flesh is carried around the entire waist. The stout individual must work twice as hard as his slim neighbor if he expects to accomplish the same object, namely, a trim, square waist.

The same exercises that reduce the waist will build it up. This applies practically to every part of the body as well. A well-developed waistline is something everyone should strive for, as the prolonged efforts utilized to obtain waist symmetry will benefit and strengthen the digestive system, and make every organ function efficiently.

Exercise 1

One of the finest exercises for the waist is to lie on the floor and come to a sitting posture, while keeping the hands behind the head. The beginner may have to hook his feet under a dresser, couch or some other piece of furniture at first, to hold his feet down, but after a while he will be able to do this exercise without any difficulty.

The exercise should be continued until the muscles in the front part of the abdomen begin to feel uncomfortable. No special rules limiting the number of repetitions can be stipulated, because everyone is constituted differently, and too severe a strain upon the waist may cause hernia and other disagreeable strains; therefore, I do not advise the student to attempt to pick up weights while performing these exercises, or sitting up with these weights until he is well advanced in the work.

I suggest that the beginner do not attempt to perform more than ten repetitions for the first week or so, increasing gradually, until about twenty-five counts are reached. When he can do twenty-five repetitions after several months, he may pick up small objects of a few pounds or more, and perform this movement.

Exercise 2

Lie on your right side and raise both legs upwards as high as possible, with the knees stiff. Lower the legs to the floor and repeat. This exercise is of special benefit for the sides of the waist, and should be performed until these waist muscles feel uncomfortable and start to ache. Do the same while lying on the opposite side.

Exercise 3

Lie on the back, and with knees stiff bring the legs as far as possible to the left, then upward as far as possible, then over to the right, until they almost touch the floor, then to the original starting position. This is called "leg circling," and is performed until the abdominal muscles feel uncomfortable. If you become tired, rest a minute and reverse the movement, until you become tired again.

Exercise 4

Raise the legs with knees stiff, and the arms with arms stiff, and touch the toe in midair while lying on your back. Lower to original position and repeat. Care should be taken each time when lowering that the body is completely outstretched on the floor, with the legs stiff and the hands extended overhead, otherwise, you will not get as much benefit out of this movement as you should. Continue until the abdominal muscles feel uncomfortable.

Exercise 5

While lying on your back, raise both legs upward and continue the movement until the toes touch the floor beyond your head. Return to original position and repeat until the abdominal region feels uncomfortable.

Exercise 6

While standing on the floor, raise arms overhead, and interlace the fingers, reaching upward as far as possible. While stretching in this position, bend as far as you can to the right, then as far as you can to the left. Continue until you feel tired at the sides of the waist or in the small of the back.

Exercise 7

Stand erect and reach upward as far as possible and clasp one hand with the other. Bend forward, keeping knees stiff, until your hands touch the floor. Raise upward again and bend backward as far as possible. These forward and backward movements you will find very suitable for warming- up exercises, before beginning heavier work.

If the student will perform the exercises I have mentioned here, he will secure about all the abdominal work necessary for his day's drill. I do not believe in devoting too much time to the abdominal muscles, for if this is done, too much energy is used, thereby preventing attention to the muscle-building exercises, which are the subject of this book.

The abdominal muscles are exercised in conjunction with various other muscles in different exercises. However, direct application to abdominal movements is absolutely essential for health's sake, as well as in cases where superfluous flesh is carried around the waist, or where greater abdominal development is desired.

The student should do at least one or two abdominal exercises every day, such as sitting up, touching the toes, or sitting up with hands behind head in order to prevent any chance of superfluous flesh gathering around his waistline, and also to stimulate his internal organs.

There is one thing I would like to emphasize before leaving this subject. The abdominal muscle exercises, above all others, are the one form of exercise you should never give up. For the older you get the more need you'll have for doing everything in your power to keep the abdominal organs functioning properly. And these are the exercises that will do the trick.

Symmetrical Hips and How to Acquire Them

Very little attention is generally paid to the hips by the average athlete in his course of training, owing to the fact that the formation of the male hips are of little consequence as far as personal pride is concerned.

If a boy or a young man should seem to show any particular interest in his hips, as an ordinary thing "the gang" would be inclined to kid the life out of him. This should not be so, because the hips are a very important element in the make-up of an athlete.

The hips vary greatly in appearance, and considerable attention should be devoted to them, because strong hips, with plenty of endurance, are a great asset to an individual. A person with wide hips naturally has a wide waist and a very strong framework and, therefore, is capable of great supporting and feats of strength in which strong hips play an important part.

The narrow-hipped individual, with a narrow waist, can never expect to be as strong, when it comes to displaying feats of strength and lifting, as his larger-framed competitor.

A person with wide hips usually has a good leg development, owing to the size and strength of his bones, and it is these individuals who, with proper scientific training, turn out to be not only the finest built athletes, but remarkably strong men as well.

Well-developed hips are essential, first, for endurance, as in running, walking, carrying heavy objects, climbing, etc., for it is in this part of the body that the first signs of fatigue are manifested in performing any of these exercises. The gluteus maximus, the largest muscle of the hip, when properly developed, gives a pleasing curve to the lower back, which is much more desirable than to see flabby tissue covering this part.

A well-trained athlete's hips usually are slightly hollow at the sides, and when contracted the gluteus maximus muscle is clearly shown. Most of the men who are "understanders," or "bottom men," in hand-balancing acts, have thoroughly developed hips. This comes naturally to them from the work they do, causing a great strain to be placed upon the hips in supporting their partner when doing hand-to-hand work.

Undoubtedly you have seen various troupes of tumbling Arabs or Japs. Possibly you have noticed that one of them, during their act, is able to support the entire troupe, who climb and pile upon him and around him. I have seen one act in particular of this nature, where a single man supported the weight of nine other men, and still was able to take a few walking steps with this enormous weight. If this man did not have exceptionally strong hips, and if his hips were not wide enough to give him exceptionally good support, this tremendous weight would cause him to collapse.

A wide-hipped man, being a heavier-boned man, as a rule, naturally is inclined to be of a heavy type, and will weigh more when in his highly developed state than an individual whose muscles are equally as well developed, but whose hips are narrow.

Undoubtedly the finest exercise to strengthen the hips is to walk while carrying heavy objects, especially while climbing stairs.

This is a very severe exercise and should not be undertaken until after you have developed a considerable amount of strength in the muscles of the hips and thighs.

1 would suggest that you first practice stair- climbing, without carrying any weights. Let the arms hang loosely at the side, and do not try to pull yourself upstairs by holding on

to the railing, or putting your hands against the wall.

After you have practiced this for a few weeks, and your strength and wind power are sufficiently developed, you might start by carrying weights, commencing with a light weight of 10 or 15 pounds, and gradually working up to it, until you can carry 50 pounds up three or four flights of stairs without any difficulty.

A great many movements can be performed for the hips, although the ones that have special merit are lateral work, such as lying on the floor on your side and raising first one leg, and then both legs, while keeping them stiff; also while lying on your stomach endeavoring to raise both legs upward, keeping the legs stiff.

While lying on your back, by performing double leg circling, you give the hips quite a play. These circles should be made as wide as possible; that is, starting from a reclining position on your back and keeping the legs stiff, bring both feet as far as you can to the left and then upward and backward over your head, and then as far as you can to the right, until they almost touch the floor. Then return to original position. All these movements should be reversed in order to work the muscles in the opposite direction.

Another excellent exercise for developing the hips is to stand on both feet, then raise the right leg with the knee stiff to a horizontal position, where it will be at right angles out in front of the body. Swing your arms up level with your shoulders, in order to keep your balance. Then lower the leg slowly and bring it up again, as often as you can, until the hips are tired. You should not do this too quickly or with any evidence of a jerk, for it is the contraction and lift of the muscles, and not the momentum of the swing, that secures the results you are aiming at in this particular exercise.

Rest for a minute or two, and then repeat the exercise, using the left leg this time, until tired.

Then rest a while, and do this same exercise, extending the legs out to the side this time, instead of straight ahead. This is more difficult than the forward lift, and you will not be able to do it so often before becoming fatigued. However, it is very important, because it brings into play different hip muscles than are stressed in the preceding exercise. Use both legs alternately, as before.

After a short rest, stand as before, and raise the legs straight backward, bringing each leg up as high as possible and holding the position a second or two, so as to get the greatest amount of good from it.

These exercises are just as good for taking off excess fat as they are for building up solid muscle—in fact, you've got to get rid of your fat before you really can put solid muscle on.

So, if you are too fat, don't be surprised to see the size of your hips reduced within a month or so, possibly by several inches. This, however, is only preliminary to building up firm, well-developed muscle, that will be of great value to you in all feats of strength, and that will serve to give your entire body much better developed and more symmetrical lines.

If you are thin and underweight, on the other hand, you will find that, after a few weeks of these exercises, you'll be conscious of a very definite increase in development.

I emphasize this matter very strongly because a great deal depends upon your hip development, if you are to bring out the general contour of your figure, and have the symmetrical lines of a perfect athlete.

The Well-Developed Thigh

The thighs, when properly developed, are undoubtedly the most beautiful sets of muscles of which the human body can boast. A well-rounded, highly developed pair of thighs will put a professional finished touch on any athlete.

Well-shaped thighs are most notable on all professional strong men, especially tumblers and weight lifters, for such physical work places direct application on the quadriceps extensor muscles, which constitute the group of muscles covering the entire front and sides of the thighs. Again I am forced to admit that Eugen Sandow had perhaps the finest contour of this group of muscles that I have ever seen.

However, the most remarkable pair of thighs, so far as size is concerned, were owned by William Gerardi, whose thighs measure, I believe, over 31 inches.

Sprinters have exceptionally developed thighs, produced by the heavy exertion of their speedy work. However, endurance runners, as a rule, are lacking greatly in leg development, as the muscles are overworked. Consequently the tissues are destroyed faster than they can be replenished. It is a known and proven fact that prolonged repetition of movement, when carried to the point of absolute fatigue and even beyond that, to exhaustion, causes the muscles to wear away. Therefore, many well- developed athletes are now dead from the effects of prolonged fatiguing exercises.

The student need have no fear, however, or be frightened by the above statement, for the strength of the muscles will be ever on the increase, as long as he discontinues the movement when the aching point is reached. At this point you should thoroughly relax and allow the blood to flow freely while in this relaxed state. After a short period of rest, resume your work until the muscles ache again, thus tiring them for the second time during the exercise period. In this way you will make most rapid progress.

The kind of exercise that the thighs are called upon to perform has a great deal to do with the size and shape of the muscles to be developed. I have found from experience that slow, heavy work is best to develop the quadriceps extensor muscles. The position of the feet must also be taken into consideration. When the feet are placed flat on the floor with the toes pointed outward, the legs somewhat spread apart, say about 18 inches or more, and deep knee- bending is performed (whether this be done with a heavy weight on the shoulders or against some powerful resistance), the sartorius muscle is brought into play. This muscle, when developed, fills in the space usually seen in poorly developed legs under the crotch, and gives not only strength, but a pleasing curve to the inside of the thighs.

The sartorius muscle is also known as the "tailor's muscle." This term was given it owing to the practice of old-time tailors who sat on the floor, and raised themselves with legs crossed and without the help of the hands, relying only on the strength of this muscle.

The vastus internus and the vastus externus, as well as the rectus femoris are the remaining three muscles that give the curve from the knee to the hip, on the inside and on the outside of the thigh. These muscles can be developed to some extent by the common deep knee-bending exercise, but if the student desires exceptional development and extraordinary curves, he must perform this deep knee- bending exercise against a powerful resistance, or else with some heavy weight on his shoulders.

The feet should be parallel with each other when performing this exercise, for the greatest strain is placed directly upon the thighs if the heels are kept flat on the floor. If the heels are raised from the floor, the lower legs or calf muscles are required to share some of the burden.

Heredity has a lot to do with the size of the legs. Some people are naturally fortunate in having fairly well-developed legs, without any exercise whatever, while others possess legs that are exceedingly thin and ungainly. A person who inherits a good- • sized leg has everything in his favor in attempting to convert the flesh into good, solid muscle — and well-formed muscle at that.

However, a person whose legs are thin need not be discouraged, for scientifically applied exercise will give anyone the curves and the strength that he desires. Of course, the small-boned man again must not expect to obtain the strength and the bulk of his heavier-boned competitor. The fact has been proven in hundreds and hundreds of cases of small-boned athletes, whose thighs were exceptionally developed, that the small-boned man has just as much of an incentive to work for, and even more than a heavy-framed individual.

The thighs play an important part in feats of strength, and work in unison with the muscles of the hips, especially in performing lifts and in carrying and working with heavy objects. The common exercise of deep knee-bending is a very good one to begin with for improvement of the thighs. However, I would not advise its continuance except as a warming-up exercise, after a period of about three months, for then the thighs are in a state to receive heavier work.

The student should then endeavor to perform deep knee-bending on one leg, or run upstairs two or three steps at a time, thereby giving the thighs additional work. After a month or two of this, you should adopt more vigorous methods, if you expect further improvement in the thigh muscles.

One of the most sadly neglected muscles in the body is the biceps femoris, below the buttocks in the back of the thigh. This muscle contracts the leg and is an exceedingly stubborn one to develop. Sprinters as a rule are well developed in this part. But in order to develop this muscle to its limit, one has to resort to special exercises.

The lifting of heavy objects from the floor while bending over and keeping the knees stiff, and then bringing the object to the waist, while straightening up to an erect position, will place pressure upon this biceps femoris muscle. Unless this muscle is properly developed the thighs lack the finishing touches of harmonious development.

Next time you attend the theatre, pay particular attention to the acrobats, the strong men or the dancers, and if you are fortunate enough to see these men's legs either with or without tights on, you will have an excellent opportunity of noting what a vast improvement a beautiful curve behind the thigh makes in the appearance of the legs.

Classical dancing will also develop this muscle. The juggling of a weight placed on your foot and held in an upright position while lying on your back, will also develop the leg biceps. The common limbering-up exercise practiced by toe dancers, which consists in grasping the heel and raising the leg forward and upward, until the knee is stiff, will also put a strain upon this muscle, and help its development.

In practicing exercises for the thigh you must be exceedingly careful in the beginning and not put too much strain upon the legs or hips, or work with too much enthusiasm. For harmful results, such as a rupture, might come from such thoughtlessness. Progress gradually; do not be impatient and expect to see results all at once. You must never try to lift heavy objects until your legs are somewhat developed, and capable of the extra strain. Then when you do, be sure that you stand pigeon-toed; that is, with the toes inclined to turn toward each other. Never stand with the toes pointed outward when lifting heavy objects. For when the toes are pointed outward, the strain is placed mostly on the sartorius and adductor muscles, and too great a strain on these muscles may prove serious. When the toes are pointed inward, the strain is placed on the vastus internus and vastus externus muscles of this quadriceps extensor group.

As I said before, the ordinary deep knee-bending exercise is a good one for beginners to use as a limbering-up movement, but it is much too light an exercise to yield any marked results in development. It won't be long before you will be able to squat down and up hundreds of times. Instead of adding strong muscular tissues on your thighs, you will tear the tissues down quicker than they can be replenished, by overwork.

Although the thigh should really be worked similarly to the arms and shoulders; that is, tiring the extensor muscles within ten repetitions, nevertheless, caution should be used in performing leg work, owing to the fact that overstraining may result in hernia. I, therefore, suggest that the student perform at least twenty or twenty-five repetitions, in order to tire the muscles thoroughly. In order to get the quadriceps extensor muscles aching in twenty- five counts, artificial resistance must be resorted to.

The best means of securing additional resistance for these exercises is to place a bar-bell upon the shoulders. Perform the deep knee-bending exercises with this weight adjusted to suit the strength of your legs. If you are good for twenty-five repetitions, and your muscles do not ache as^much as they did in the beginning, you should increase the weight. If you have no weight I suggest you perform the deep knee-bending exercise on one leg at a time. In this manner, you will be able to tire your muscles more readily.

To make the movement still more difficult without the use of a weight, you can step up on the edge of a table until you are standing in an erect position. Then lower yourself again, until one leg touches the floor. This gives the muscles a little more work than if you performed a one-leg deep knee-bend on the floor.

There is still another method of developing the thighs, if the student has no bar-bell. That is, to have someone sit on your shoulders, straddling your neck, and perform your deep knee-bending exercise that way. Progress can be made by having heavier and heavier individuals help you out.

When performing deep knee-bending with barbell or with someone sitting on your shoulders, keep the feet flat on the floor. Do not raise the heels off the floor when reaching the squatting position. This will enable you to squat further down and almost sit on the floor, thereby giving complete contractions and extensions to your muscles. Keep your toes pointed front and your feet about 12 inches apart.

Another exercise that will greatly build up the belly of the extensor muscles and, at the same time, give strong play to the sartorius muscle, is as follows:

Stand with feet about 20 inches apart or more, depending upon the length of your legs. Then, with a weight on your shoulders, and toes pointed outward, with feet flat on the floor, perform a half- squat, that is, bend the knees about half way. This can also be done with a bar-bell held with both hands between your crotch. In performing this movement, be sure to keep the body erect and tire the muscles within twenty-five repetitions. Care should be taken by the beginner in this exercise not to use too heavy a weight or resistance. For when the toes are pointed outward, there is more danger of a strain or hernia that when the toes are pointing straight forward, or even inward.

However, you need not fear a strain if you go about it systematically and do not let your ambitions and enthusiasm get the better of you.

Almost every athlete who has well-developed legs also has an excellent lung capacity, for you cannot develop the legs without developing the lungs at the same time. You will find this out for yourself as you progress with the work. It will be a good thing to do a little breathing exercise after you have finished your leg work, for then you will be out of breath, and when you are out of breath, deep breathing will do you a world of good.

The muscle behind the thighs, known as the biceps of the legs, as I told you previously, is a sadly neglected muscle and is very seldom prominent, even on many professional athletes. There are dozens of movements that you can perform to work this muscle, but here are two of the best. Bend over with the knees stiff and pick up a heavy weight from the floor, bring it to an erect position in front of you, and lower again. Repeat this until the muscles at the back of the legs are distinctly tired. Lie on your stomach, bending your knees until your heels almost touch your hips, and push one leg with the other until your legs are straight, forcing yourself to work against as much resistance as your legs will permit.

Also, in picking up a bar-bell from the floor, exercise should be made progressive as you become stronger in the leg biceps, by standing on books or low stools and picking the weights up from the floor, with the knees stiff. If you bend your knees at all in this exercise, you lose the most important part of it.

By keeping the knees stiff at all times, you will feel the strain directly upon the biceps of the legs. The simple exercise of bending over and touching the floor with the palms of your hands, without bending your knees, also affects this muscle, but you will not make much progress by continuing this light movement. You should progress in this exercise until you are able to stand on a strong chair that will not tip over, and with the bar-bell held in front of you, bend over with knees stiff until the weight hangs down below your feet as far as possible, and then straighten up again as far as possible. By adjusting the resistance you work against, you should very easily tire your leg biceps muscle within twenty-five repetitions, or even less.

In the exercise where you lie on your stomach and resist with your legs, you must concentrate strongly on this movement.

Otherwise, the amount of resistance you work against will become lighter and lighter, in which case you will not progress very rapidly.

Lying on your back and juggling a bar-bell placed on your feet when your feet are extended upward, will also benefit this muscle. But I do not advise this exercise except to advanced students who have become used to handling a bar-bell. For the beginner is liable to allow the bell to slip off his feet and fall on him, thereby resulting in an injury.

Short sprints will also benefit the thigh muscles, for they put direct strain on these muscles and give them definite work to do. However, as I said when speaking of the hips—and the same thing applies to the thighs—if you want to be a developed athlete, with a well-rounded physique, perfect in all its proportions, don't neglect your hips and thighs. For lack of care in exercising these muscles will be apparent, at first glance, to any trainer or teacher of physical culture, and will inevitably detract from the harmonious appearance your body would otherwise have.

The Calf and Its Sturdy Curve

A short time ago I was at a gathering at which there were several famous stage beauties, who were known for their devotion to physical culture. The discussion naturally turned toward physical culture and its influence on health and beauty, which was admitted by everybody.

Finally, one of the ladies, known to every theatregoer for her wonderful ability as a dancer, turned to me and said:

"Mr. Liederman, there's one thing that has always impressed me on the bathing beaches. There isn't one man in a thousand who hasn't ugly legs. Either they are too fat, or they are too stringy and skinny.

"You may see hundreds of girls with beautifully formed legs, calves and ankles, but you very seldom see a man who would pass muster, especially from his knees down. Why is this?"

I replied that very few men pay any attention to symmetrical development, or muscle building. They try to build up a big chest, or shoulders or arms. But they hardly ever give a thought to their lower extremities. These leg muscles do not show so much for the work put in on their development. Again, the means used to bring about this development are practically unknown, except to a few physical culture specialists—who have paid particular attention to building up these ordinarily stringy muscles into well-rounded proportions.

As a matter of fact, the calf of the leg is, without doubt, one of the hardest parts of the body to develop, owing to the fact that the muscle is continually placed in a contracted state by walking, and the further fact that it responds very slowly to exercise. The size and shape of the calf, the same as with the thigh, depends greatly upon heredity. Some people fortunately possess well-shaped legs below the knee, while others less fortunate have great difficulty in developing the muscles of the calf even to fair proportions.

A person with an exceptionally developed pair of calves, regardless of what some people may claim, must, in the first place, have had a certain amount of fleshy tissue to begin with. Then, with considerable muscle-building work, he will be able to develop the gastrocnemius muscle behind the calf to exceptional proportions.

Again, the length of the bone must be taken into consideration. The tall individual with long bones cannot develop a calf in proportion to a chap whose legs are short. Therefore, you usually find phenomenal calf development among people of somewhat short stature. In order to give his calves the proper amount of attention the lanky individual has to do double the amount of work that the fellow who begins with a little beef in this part of his anatomy has to do.

The common exercise of rising up and down on the toes will start the student off with calf development. However, he cannot expect to develop to any marked degree by this light exercise. Therefore, after a few weeks, he should resort to rising up and down on the toes on one leg at a time. He will then have to progress again after a short period by working the calves against a stronger resistance, and keep on progressing.

The calves should be tired at least two or three times during each exercise period. The student need have little fear of overstraining the muscles of the calf, because they are capable of supporting great strain.

The calves are one of the first places varicose veins put in their appearance. These are caused by continual standing on the feet, thereby keeping the muscles in an over-tensed state, and consequently causing the walls of the veins and arteries to become weakened.

To the average student the gastrocnemius muscle, or the muscle behind the calf, constitutes the main object of lower leg development. In reality, however, a muscle of vital importance is the muscle of the shin, for this muscle, when properly developed, gives the calf 50 per cent, more attention value, and changes the appearance of the outside and front of the calf.

The size of the ankle has a great deal to do with the shape of the calf. A person who has small ankles will undoubtedly have better shaped legs than a person whose ankles are thick and heavy. It is a peculiar thing, and one that very few people seem to know anything about, but persons with thick ankles are usually subject to weak ankles. The slim-ankled individual hardly ever develops sprains or strains in this part.

Much of what I have said regarding the development of the muscles of the thighs and the hips applies with almost equal force to the calves. Running, jumping, and climbing are especially valuable. I also recommend rope skipping, especially when you spring from the toes with each skip, as this puts direct strain on the muscle of the calf.

It goes without saying that this exercise is also splendid for lung development and for increasing wind and endurance. I also recommend dancing as a good exercise for developing the calves, especially if you'll "stay up on your toes" as much as you can, and not slouch into the lazy habit of spending most of your time on the soles of your feet.

I do not believe it is possible to over-emphasize the importance of development of the muscles of the calves in bringing about a more springy and elastic stride when walking, and even a moderate amount of weakness or lack of development in the calf muscles will diminish the grace and freedom of your walk. This springiness is one of the first things you lose when the arches of your feet break down. And the lack of the power and development that brings about this springiness, is in turn one of the chief evidences of that relaxation of the muscles that finally results in flat feet.

So remember that whatever exercise you are practicing to develop the muscles of the calves, it will also help strengthen the muscles of the arches of the feet.

As the calves of the legs are so hard to develop, owing to constant walking, the student should not become discouraged if the progress is much slower than in other parts of his body. However, the simple rising up and down on his toes will develop the gastrocnemius muscle behind the upper calf to a certain extent. But better progress can be made if this exercise is performed on one leg at a time and the muscle is tired within twenty or twenty-five repetitions.

Still better results can be accomplished by rising up and down on the toes with the weight of a barbell, or a progressive exerciser that offers similar resistance. Further and quicker progress still can be made by performing this exercise against artificial resistance, with the toes resting on a book, thus giving the gastrocnemius muscle more play.

When the student eventually discovers that this last exercise is becoming too light for him, he can perform it on one leg at a time.

The shin muscle, called the tibialis anticus, really makes up the contour of the leg, when properly developed and when viewed from the front, for this muscle presents a pleasing curve to the anterior portion of the calf. It is developed by keeping the feet flat on the floor and bending the knees forward as far as possible, without raising the heels from the floor.

If you will perform this movement with a barbell on your shoulder, or with someone sitting on your shoulder, you will soon observe a different appearance to your calves. Sprinting will again prove an important factor in the development of the calves, although you should limit your sprints to 100 yards at the most. Sprinting is a great developer for the calves, but endurance running is not. For, as I have mentioned previously, endurance runners usually have thin legs, while sprinters are well knotted up and symmetrically developed.

In order to get the most complete development of your calves, I would suggest that you secure a block of wood, or a good thick book that will raise you about four inches from the floor. Stand on this with the heels, the toes extending over the edge of the block of wood or book and touching the floor. Now raise the toes as high as you can, using the utmost strain possible. Relax and then repeat until you are tired. This is splendid for the flexor muscles on the anterior or front of the lower leg.

Then stand on the external edge of the book on your toes, and allow yourself to drop down as far as possible. Then raise slowly as far as you can, let yourself drop back, and repeat the exercise until you have a very definite ache in the muscles of the back, or posterior portion of the calf.

Now stand with the toes resting on the book, and roll the feet until the entire weight of the body rests on the outer sides of the feet. Then roll back again until the weight of the body rests on the inner sides of the feet. Repeat this exercise until the muscles in the inside and the outside of your calves feel tired.

You will find that these exercises will develop every muscle in the lower leg, and with such symmetry and uniformity that the calves will be in perfect proportion, and you will possess something that few men ever take the trouble to develop—a shapely and muscular pair of calves.